COPYCAT RECIPE

HOW TO MAKE PANERA BREAD RECIPES AT HOME

PATTY STEWART

Edition 2020

© Copyright 2019 by – All rights reserved

This document is geared towards providing exact and reliable information in regards to the topic and issue covered. The publication is sold with the idea that the publisher is not required to render accounting, officially permitted, or otherwise, qualified services. If advice is necessary legal or professional, a practiced individual in the profession should be ordered.

From a Declaration of Principles which was accepted and approved equally by a Committee of the American Bar Association and a Committee of Publishers and Associations.

In no way is it legal to reproduce, duplicate or transmit any part of this document in either electronic means or in oriented format. Recording of this publication is strictly prohibited and any storage of this document is not allowed unless with written permission from the publisher. All rights reserved.

The information provided herein is stated to be truthful and consistent, in that any liability, in terms of inattention or otherwise, by any usage or abuse of any policies, processes, or directions contained within is the solitary and utter responsibility of the recipient reader. Under no circumstances will any legal responsibility or blame be held against the publisher for any reparation, damages, or monetary loss due to the information herein, either directly or indirectly.

Respective authors own all copyrights not held by the publisher.

The information herein is offered for informational purposes solely, and is universal as so. The presentation of the information is without contract or any type of guarantee assurance.

The trademarks that are used are without any consent and the publication of the trademark is without permission or backing by the trademark owner. All trademarks and brands within this book are for clarifying purposes and are the owned by the owners themselves, not affiliated to with this document.

TABLE OF CONTENTS

Introduction	6
Panera Bread Copycat Baked Potato Soup	7
Panera Bread Copycat Broccoli Cheddar Soup	10
Panera Bread Copycat Creamy Tomato Soup	13
Panera Bread Copycat Bistro French Onion Soup	16
Panera Bread Copycat Autumn Squash Soup	19
Panera Bread Copycat Black Bean Soup	22
Panera Bread Copycat Macaroni and Cheese	25
Panera Bread Copycat Green Goddess Cobb Salad	28
Panera Bread Copycat Steak & Cheddar White Panini	32
Panera Bread Copycat Panini Bread	35
Panera Bread Copycat Tuna Salad Sandwich	38
Panera Bread Copycat Turkey Sandwich	41
Panera Bread Copycat Pumpkin Muffin	44
Panera Bread Copycat Instant Pot Chicken And Wild Rice Soup	47
Panera Bread Copycat BBQ Chicken Salad	50

Panera bread Copycat Chocolate Chip Cookies	53
Panera Bread Copycat Chicken Noodle Soup	56
Panera Bread Copycat Spinach and Cheese Egg Souffle	59
Panera Bread Copycat Napa Almond Chicken Salad	62
Panera Bread Copycat Cranberry Orange Muffins	65
Panera Bread Copycat Chopped Thai Grilled Chicken Salad	68
Panera Bread Copycat Apple Raisin Cobblestone Muffins	72
Panera Bread Copycat Lemon Chicken Orzo Soup	76
Panera Bread Copycat Fuji Apple Salad	79
Panera Bread Copycat Green Tea	82
Panera Bread Copycat Hummus Bowl	84
Panera Bread Copycat Honey Walnut Panera Cream Cheese	88
Panera Bread Copycat Asiago cheese bread	90
Panera Bread Copycat Soba Noodle Broth Bowl with Chicken	93
Panera Bread Copycat Chicken Caesar Sandwich	96
Panera Bread Copycat Spinach and Artichoke Souffle	99
Panera Bread Copycat Bacon Turkey Bravo Sandwich	102
Panera Bread Copycat Cream Cheese Potato Soup	105
Panera Bread Copycat Frontega Chicken Panini	107
Panera Bread Copycat Orange Scones	110

Panera Bread Copycat Asian Sesame Chicken Salad	113
Panera Bread Copycat Brown Betty	116
Harvest Turkey Salad with Cherry Vinaigrette	119
Panera Bread Copycat Chipotle Chicken Avocado Melt	123
Panera Bread Copycat Modern Greek Salad	126
Panera Bread Menu	129
Conclusion	144

INTRODUCTION

Everyone loves a good recipe from their favorite restaurant. One of my favorites seems to be Panera. They have incredibly delicious soups, salads, and bread. Panera copycat recipes are fun to recreate, saving you money and making bigger portions, so you can enjoy them multiple times at home instead of just in the restaurant.

Panera bread is known for having excellent soups, salads, sandwiches, desserts, and of course, bagels. The casual and fast restaurant offers excellent classic dishes and seasonal cuisine that are good all year round. Well, thanks to this Panera Bread Copycat Recipes guide, you can make any of these delicacies at home!

These are Panera Bread Copycat recipes for everything from soups to desserts. These recipes are easy to prepare in your home kitchen, even without much kitchen experience. Forget the stress of having to go to Panera Bread restaurants for lunch every day and create your own Panera delicacy right at home. Be sure to save some of the Panera Copycat dessert recipes because these treats will be a huge success the next time you have guests.

From broccoli and cheese soup to your favorite BBQ chicken salad, I have compiled 40 of the tastiest Panera Bread recipes that are sure to make you drool and the perfect way to get those comforting meals right at home.

PANERA BREAD COPYCAT BAKED POTATO SOUP

Baked Potato Soup with Bread Loaf is a wonderful creamy soup that will warm your soul. It is filled with potato wedges, cream cheese, and smoked bacon wedges. You will soon fall in love with this recipe.

Total time: 30 minutes
Yield: 6 Servings

INGREDIENTS

- 2 teaspoons of chicken soup base
- 4 cups low-sodium chicken broth
- 1/2 white onion, chopped
- 2 kilos of rubbed, peeled and diced potatoes
- 2 butter spoons
- 1 teaspoon minced garlic
- 4 ounces cream cheese
- 2 tablespoons of flour
- 1/2 teaspoon black pepper
- 1/2 teaspoon salt
- 2 tablespoons of bacon
- 2 teaspoons of chives

INSTRUCTIONS

- In a medium saucepan, add the chopped potatoes, chicken stock, and soup base. Cook the potatoes in broth over medium heat for about 12-15 minutes or until the potatoes are tender when pricked with a fork.

- In a large saucepan, heat the butter until it melts over medium heat, add the brown, onions and garlic until the onions are translucent.

- Sprinkle the flour with the butter and cook for at least 1 minute. The flour and butter mixture should become fragrant. Add the chicken and potato stock in 1-cup increments and stir until the soup mixture is well blended.

- Continue until all potatoes and broth are added. Add cream cheese and stir until dissolved. Add salt, black pepper, chives, and pieces of bacon. If desired, garnish the soup with grated cheese, bacon bits, and sour cream.

Take your Notes Here and Create your Variant

PANERA BREAD COPYCAT BROCCOLI CHEDDAR SOUP

This creamy broccoli cheddar soup is excellent for a hearty lunch. It's easy to make - just have frozen broccoli, fresh carrots, and two types of cheese to make this soup.

Total Time: 40 minutes
Yield: 6 Servings

INGREDIENTS

- 2 tablespoons all-purpose flour
- 2 butter spoons
- 1 cup half and half
- 1/2 cup chopped white onion
- 8 ounces shredded cheddar cheese
- 16 ounces American Velveeta cheese
- 16 ounces frozen chopped broccoli
- 29 ounces low-sodium chicken broth 2 cans
- 1 cup carrots, sliced or diced Julianne
- Salt and pepper to taste

INSTRUCTIONS

- In a large saucepan, melt the butter. Mix the flour and the onion. Cook for at least 1 minute, then slowly add half and half, about 1/4 cup at a time, whisking until it becomes smooth and thick.

- When half and half are incorporated, add broccoli and melted cheese.

- Once the cheese melts completely, add the chicken stock 1 cup at a time, occasionally stirring, until the soup is well mixed and has a consistent consistency. Add carrots and simmer for about 10 minutes.

- Mix the cheddar and cook for another 10 minutes. Season with salt and pepper to taste. Serve when all the cheese is completely melted and mixed.

Take your Notes Here and Create your Variant

PANERA BREAD COPYCAT CREAMY TOMATO SOUP

You'll love this creamy vegetarian tomato soup that tastes of Panera. Enjoy your bowl of Panera creamy tomato soup, even more, when you make it at home.

Total time: 30 minutes
Yield: 8 servings

INGREDIENTS

- 1 cup chopped white onion
- 2 tablespoons of olive oil
- 1/2 teaspoon salt
- 2 teaspoons dried basil
- 58 ounces tomato sauce 4 - 14.5 ounces cans
- 2 teaspoons minced garlic
- 14.5 ounces vegetable broth
- 1/2 teaspoon oregano
- 1 teaspoon of sugar
- 1/2 cup of cream
- Black pepper and salt to taste

INSTRUCTIONS

- In a large saucepan over medium heat, add the olive oil and add the chopped white onion. Sprinkle 1/2 teaspoon of salt on top. Sauté until the onions are transparent.
- Add minced garlic and sauté until garlic becomes fragrant.
- Add the tomato puree, basil, oregano, vegetable stock and cream. Reduce heat to low heat. Boil for about 10-15 minutes.
- Try it and if the soup is too sour, add sugar. Season with salt and black pepper to taste.
- Puree soup with an immersion blender or mix soup well in a blender.

Take your Notes Here and Create your Variant

PANERA BREAD COPYCAT BISTRO FRENCH ONION SOUP

Panera Bread Bistro French Onion Soup has been removed from the menu and is now back. Enjoy a bowl of Bistro French Onion Soup at home.

Total time: 55 minutes
Yield: 8 Servings

INGREDIENTS

- 4 kilos of chopped yellow onion
- 4 tablespoons of butter
- 1 tablespoon of flour
- 1 teaspoon salt
- 14.5 ounces chicken broth
- 1 cup croutons
- 32 ounces beef broth
- 2 tablespoons beef base
- 1/2 teaspoon thyme
- 1/4 cup grated Gruyère cheese
- Cheese Mix
- 1 tablespoon of Asiago cheese

INSTRUCTIONS

- In a large saucepan over medium-high heat, add the chopped onion and butter. Add 1 teaspoon of salt to the onions. Fry the onions for about 20 minutes or until golden.

- Add 1 tablespoon of flour and stir to coat the flour onions. Bake, the flour for another minute or until it, becomes as fragrant as the tart crust.

- Add beef broth, chicken broth, beef base, and thyme. Reduce heat to low temperature. Cook the soup for another 15-20 minutes. Before serving the top with croutons and grated cheeses.

Take your Notes Here and Create your Variant

PANERA BREAD COPYCAT AUTUMN SQUASH SOUP

Prepare this classic autumn soup at any time with this recipe. Autumn squash soup is a seasonal offer; you can prepare it throughout the year.

Total time: 1 hour
Yield: 10 Servings

INGREDIENTS

- 2 tablespoons divided-use vegetable oil
- 1 cup chopped white onion
- 2 pounds of butternut squash
- 2 cups of vegetable broth
- 15 ounces pumpkin
- 1/2 teaspoon of cinnamon
- 2 teaspoons of curry powder you may want to add more
- 1 tablespoon of honey
- 1 cup apple juice
- 1 tablespoon of pumpkin seeds
- 1/2 cup of cream

INSTRUCTIONS

- Preheat oven to 350 degrees. Peel and slice a 1 inch diced pumpkin pie. Pour 1 tablespoon of vegetable oil over the pumpkin and mix to coat it well. Bake for at least 30 minutes or until the squash is tender. Don't let the pumpkin turn brown.

- In a large saucepan, add 1 tablespoon of vegetable oil and fry the onions until translucent.

- Sprinkle a little salt on the onions as you toss them. By salting the onions, you will get the moisture from the onions and the onions will cook faster.

- When the onions are translucent, add pumpkin, squash, vegetable broth, curry and apple juice, cinnamon, and honey. Then heat.

- When hot, use an immersion blender to soften the soup. If desired, you can use a blender to prepare the soup. Add cream to the soup and mix the cream.

- Toast the pumpkin seeds in a small skillet. Heat until fragrant. Immediately remove from heat.

Take your Notes Here and Create your Variant

PANERA BREAD COPYCAT BLACK BEAN SOUP

This Black Bean Soup is a vegetarian soup full of genuine ingredients that you will love. Try making this at home and enjoy it with the rest of your family.

Total time: 40 minutes
Yield: 8 Servings

INGREDIENTS

- 1/2 cup chopped celery
- 1 cup chopped white onion
- 2 tablespoons of vegetable oil
- 1/2 cup carrot, chopped
- 2 teaspoons minced garlic
- 1/2 cup chopped red bell pepper
- 30 ounces black beans or 3-4 cups cooked black beans
- 32 ounces vegetable broth
- 1-2 teaspoons of cumin
- 1-2 teaspoons of salt
- 1 tablespoon cornstarch mixed with 1 tablespoon water
- 1 1/2 teaspoon lemon juice

INSTRUCTIONS

- In a large saucepan, add 2 tablespoons of vegetable oil. Fry the onions, celery and carrots. Sprinkle the vegetables with a pinch of salt to help release the water in the vegetables.
- When the onions start to become translucent, add pepper and garlic. Continue sautéing the vegetables until the garlic becomes fragrant.
- If you use canned black beans, rinse them to remove excess starch. Add beans and vegetable stock to the pot. Add 1 teaspoon of salt and cumin to the soup. Let the soup cook for about 10 minutes to heat it up.
- Try the soup and, if necessary, adjust the salt. Add the cornstarch and water mixture to the soup. It will help thicken the soup. Just before serving, add the lemon juice.

TAKE YOUR NOTES HERE AND CREATE YOUR VARIANT

PANERA BREAD COPYCAT MACARONI AND CHEESE

Panera Bread Macaroni and cheese must be one of my favorite dishes at Panera Bread. It is rich, creamy and irresistible.

Total Time: 25 minutes
Yield: 10 Servings

INGREDIENTS

- 3 tablespoons of butter
- 1 pasta shell
- 2 cups of milk
- 2 teaspoons Dijon mustard
- 3 tablespoons of flour
- 1/4 pound of grated white cheddar cheese
- 3/4 pounds of American white cheese

INSTRUCTIONS

- Prepare the pasta according to the package instructions. Prepare the sauce while the pasta cooks.
- Prepare a basic white sauce by first of all melting the 3 tablespoons of butter, mix with flour and cook for about 1 minute over medium heat. Then slowly add the cold milk

and stir the sauce until it thickens.

- Add the American white cheese to the bechamel sauce. If the American white cheese is not sliced, cut it into cubes.
- In the medium saucepan, add the American cheese and when it begins to melt, slowly add the milk.
- Once the American cheese has completely melted, begin mixing the sharp white cheese. Add Dijon mustard. The cheese sauce must be ready at the same time as the pasta. Combine the cheese and pasta together. Serve immediately

Take your Notes Here and Create your Variant

PANERA BREAD COPYCAT GREEN GODDESS COBB SALAD

This salad is perfect for keto and low carb diets (just remove the pickled onions). Best of all, Green Goddess Panera Bread's Cobb salads don't taste like a diet. This is a salad that many people love.

Total time: 20 minutes
Yield: 2 servings

INGREDIENTS

Pickled Onions

- 1 cup sliced red onion
- 1 spoon of sugar
- 1/2 cup of white vinegar
- 1 cup hot water
- 1 1/2 teaspoons of salt

Assemble the salad

- 3 tablespoons chopped avocado
- 2 tablespoons cooked crispy bacon
- 6 ounces grilled chicken breast
- 6-ounce salad mix with arugula, romaine lettuce, black cabbage, and chicory mixture

- 1 cooked egg cut in half
- 1/2 cup of chopped tomatoes
- 2 tablespoons of pickled onion
- 2 tablespoons of feta cheese

Green Goddess Salad Dressing

- 2 tablespoons of tarragon leaves
- 1 cup mayonnaise
- 1 cup flat-leaf parsley
- 3 tablespoons chopped chives
- 2 tablespoons of lemon juice
- 1/4 teaspoon of pepper
- 1 cup clean watercress and hard stems removed
- 1/2 teaspoon salt
- 1 tablespoon of champagne vinegar

INSTRUCTIONS

Pickled Onions

- Cut the onions as thin as possible, I like to use the 1/8 inch setting on my mandolin. Put the onions in a distant glass.
- In a small bowl, mix the white vinegar, sugar, salt, and hot water. Stir until sugar and salt dissolve. These should rest about 30 minutes for use.

Green Goddess Salad Dressing

- Put all the seasoning ingredients in the bowl of a blender or food processor and stir for at least 30 seconds, or until the salad dressing is creamy and smooth.

Assemble the salad

- Place the salad in the bottom of a large salad bowl. Cut the chicken breast into thin slices and put it on the lettuce.
- Add the bacon, chopped avocado, chopped tomatoes, feta cheese, half the hard-boiled egg, and pickled onions.
- Sprinkle with all desired salad dressing. The remaining salad dressing can be stored in an airtight container for 1 week.

TAKE YOUR NOTES HERE AND CREATE YOUR VARIANT

PANERA BREAD COPYCAT STEAK & CHEDDAR WHITE PANINI

Pickled purple onions are the secret to this yummy Panera bread specialty. Enjoy the Panera Bread Steak & White Cheddar Panini at home.

Total time: 15 minutes
Yield: 2 servings

INGREDIENTS

Pickled red onions

- 1/2 cup of white vinegar
- 1 cup red onion, thinly sliced
- 1 1/2 teaspoons of salt
- 1 cup hot water
- 1 spoon of sugar

Sandwich

- 2 tablespoons of pickled red onion
- 4 slices of white cheddar cheese
- 1 loaf of ciabatta bread
- 6 ounces sliced roast beef

- 2 tablespoons horseradish sauce
- Cooking spray for the frying pan

INSTRUCTIONS

Pickled White Onions

- Cut the onions as thin as possible; I like to use the 1/8 inch setting on my mandolin. Put the onions in a glass jar.
- In a small bowl, combine the white vinegar, sugar, salt, and hot water. Stir until sugar and salt dissolve.
- Pour the liquid into the jar with the onions. These should rest about 30 minutes for use.

Sandwich

- Divide the open ciabatta bread, distribute the horseradish sauce on top inside the divided bread. Add roast beef to the bottom. Add the cheese and pickled onions.
- Place in the press and cook for about 3 minutes or until the sandwich is heated.
- Heat up the Panini press. If you don't have a sandwich press, you can use a roasting pan and a heavy object to compress the sandwich in the pan. You can also wrap a brick with a sheet of paper and use it as a press.

TAKE YOUR NOTES HERE AND CREATE YOUR VARIANT

PANERA BREAD COPYCAT PANINI BREAD

This soft, chewy bread is the best bread for making sandwiches; If it is filled with red peppers in tomato oil and cooked on the grill, it is an ideal lunch or dinner.

Total time: 33 minutes
Yield: 12 Servings (12 loaves)

INGREDIENTS

Starter/Biga

- 250 grams of flour
- 140 ml of water
- 2 g yeast

PANINI BREAD DOUGH

- 10 grams of salt
- 500 grams of flour
- 10 grams of honey
- 25 grams of olive oil
- 50 grams of sun-dried tomatoes
- 300 ml of water

- 12 g yeast

INSTRUCTIONS

- Start by creating the starter culture. Mix everything indicated under the starter ingredients and combine to form a dough. It is not necessary to knead the dough here. Just stir to form a dough. Wrap and leave to ferment overnight or at least 8 hours.
- The next day to make the dough, take the flour, salt, olive oil, honey and the cart in the mixer. Dissolve yeast in water and add it to the food processor. Knead the dough for 8 minutes.
- After 8 minutes, add the sun-dried tomato and mix for another 30 seconds.
- Lightly oil the bowl and transfer the paste to the bowl and let it taste for 40 minutes.
- After 40 minutes, resize and round the dough to 100 grams each and allow a 10-minute intermediate correction.
- Then take a round, crush it, and shape it into a torpedo. (See the paragraph above for a graphic representation or watch the video) Using a rolling pin simply flatten them to give a palm-sized oval shape.
- Line it up on a baking sheet previously lined with parchment paper. Let stand for 10 minutes and then bake in a preheated oven at 160 ° C for 14-18 minutes.
- Let it cool completely before slicing, filling, and roasting your favorite sandwich.

Take your Notes Here and Create your Variant

PANERA BREAD COPYCAT TUNA SALAD SANDWICH

Prepare this Panera Tuna sandwich at home and save your trip to the restaurant. A simple recipe for tuna salad served on wheat slices.

Total time: 15 minutes
Yield: 4 Servings

INGREDIENTS

- 1 1/2 teaspoon mayonnaise
- 1 can of drained tuna
- 3/4 teaspoon Dijon mustard
- 8 slices of wholemeal honey bread
- 1 teaspoon of sweet dressing
- Red onion slices
- Sliced tomatoes
- Salt and pepper to taste

INSTRUCTIONS

- Mix the tuna, mayonnaise, seasoning, and mustard in a bowl.
- Store in the refrigerator for at least 10 minutes.

- Serve on whole-wheat bread with leaf lettuce, red onion slice, and sliced tomato.

Take your Notes Here and Create your Variant

PANERA BREAD COPYCAT TURKEY SANDWICH

This turkey sandwich is the best! Roasted turkey, sweet apple slices, and sharp cheddar are sandwiched between homemade cranberry walnut bread.

Total time: 5 minutes
Yield: 4 servings

INGREDIENTS

- 4 ounces sliced sharp white cheddar cheese
- 8-10 ounces thickly sliced roasted turkey breast
- 8 slices of cranberry walnut bread
- 1 gala apple, thinly sliced (or another sweet apple)
- 1/2 red onion cut into thin slices
- 8 pieces of bread-size lettuce

Homemade honey mustard

- 3 tablespoons Dijon mustard
- 1 tablespoon of honey

INSTRUCTIONS

- Prepare honey and mustard by mixing honey and mustard.

Distribute on the 8 slices of bread.

- Layer 4 slices of bread with turkey, apple, cheese, onion and lettuce. Place the remaining 4 slices of bread on the sandwiches and cut them. Serve immediately

Take your Notes Here and Create your Variant

PANERA BREAD COPYCAT PUMPKIN MUFFIN

Panera Pumpkin Muffins are easy to make and wettest jumbo pumpkin muffins with quick crumb topping.

Total time: 55 minutes
Yield: 3 servings (6 cupcakes)

INGREDIENTS

Crumb toppings:

- 2 tablespoons of granulated sugar
- 1 tablespoon of vegetable oil
- 1/3 cup all-purpose flour
- 1/4 teaspoon of cinnamon
- 2 teaspoons of honey

Toppings:

- Powdered sugar

Muffin:

- 2 teaspoons of baking powder
- 1 3/4 cups all-purpose flour

- 1/2 teaspoon salt
- 1/3 cup vegetable oil
- 2 eggs
- 2 teaspoons of spices per pumpkin pie
- 1 cup pumpkin (not filled with pumpkin pie)
- 1 1/4 cups granulated sugar

INSTRUCTIONS

- Preheat oven to about 375 degrees F. Line a giant muffin tin with 6 paper bags.
- Prepare the crumb stamp. Mix 1/3 cup flour, cinnamon, 2 tablespoons sugar, honey, and 1 tablespoon vegetable oil in a small bowl until small crumbs form, then set aside.
- In a bigger bowl, mix 1 1/4 cups flour, pumpkin pie spices, baking powder, and salt until well blended.
- Mix 1/3 cup oil, 1 1/4 cups sugar, pumpkin, and 2 eggs together with a whisk or large spoon in a medium bowl until it is well mixed.
- Pour the mixture over the flour mixture and mix until combined. Put the muffin dough in the prepared skillet. Sprinkle crumbs over the muffins.
- Bake the muffins at 375 degrees F for about 25-30 minutes or until the golden brown around the edges and the toothpick inserted in the middle are clean.
- Cool slightly, then remove the muffins from the pan and place them on the wire rack to finish cooling. When completely cold, sprinkle lightly with icing sugar.

Take your Notes Here and Create your Variant

PANERA BREAD COPYCAT INSTANT POT CHICKEN AND WILD RICE SOUP

This is one of my favorite Panera bread recipes. Prepare this instant pot chicken and wild rice soup at home and save your trip to the restaurant.

Total time: 35 minutes
Yield: 6 servings

INGREDIENTS

- 32 ounces chicken broth
- 2 large chicken breasts
- 1 cup celery, chopped
- 1 4.3-ounce box wild Roni rice
- 1 chopped onion
- 2 tablespoons of olive oil
- 1 clove garlic
- 1 cup of cream or milk
- 1 teaspoonful of oregano
- 1 teaspoon of basil

INSTRUCTIONS

- Put the instant pot on fry, add oil, garlic, onion and

vegetables in the instant pot.
- Add chicken (mine was frozen).
- Add chicken stock, rice, and seasoning pack.
- Add basil and oregano.
- Set the pot to 30 minutes at high pressure manually or just use the soup button
- Take a quick pitch.
- Remove the chicken and the strips.
- Add it to your soup.
- Put the pan in the pan.
- Mix 1 cup broth with 2 tablespoons cornstarch to create a suspension.
- Pour in cream and grout; continue to sauté until thick.
- Note that it thickens more as it is. Enjoy!

Take your Notes Here and Create your Variant

PANERA BREAD COPYCAT BBQ CHICKEN SALAD

This Panera Copycat barbecue chicken salad recipe is a delicious suitable for both lunch and dinner. It is as healthy as it is tasty and so simple and fast that it practically begs you to do it for a simple week-long dinner!

Total time: 10 minutes
Yield: 2 servings

INGREDIENTS

- Tomatoes cut into small pieces.
- Chopped lettuce
- Grilled chicken breast, sliced (or any leftover chicken)
- Roasted corn sauce
- Barbecue sauce
- Chives, chopped
- Fried onions
- Barbecue seasoning
- 1 part barbecue sauce
- 1 part ranch sauce

INSTRUCTIONS

- Mix the lettuce, tomatoes, and corn sauce in a bowl. Set aside.
- In a small bowl, beat together the ranch dressing and barbecue sauce until well combined.
- Toss salad with ranch barbecue sauce to lightly coat.
- Add chicken, fried onions, chives, and a pinch of barbecue sauce and serve immediately.

TAKE YOUR NOTES HERE AND CREATE YOUR VARIANT

PANERA BREAD COPYCAT CHOCOLATE CHIP COOKIES

The perfect cookie with oversized chocolate chips. Chewy and almost cooked in the center and perfectly crispy on the edges, these chocolate chip cookies are not much better than that.

Total time: 22 minutes
Yield: 6 Servings (18 cookies)

INGREDIENTS

- 1 1/4 cups light brown sugar
- 2 pieces of butter + 5 tablespoons softened (I used salty)
- 1 1/2 tablespoons vanilla extract
- 1/4 cup white sugar
- 1/2 teaspoon extra salt if you use unsalted butter
- 2 eggs at room temperature
- 1/4 teaspoon baking powder
- 3/4 teaspoons of baking soda
- 2 cups of chocolate chips
- 3 cups of flour

INSTRUCTIONS

- Beat the softened butter until smooth and light. Add sugar and beat 2 minutes over medium-high heat until super smooth. Add the vanilla, combine, and then add the eggs one at a time, beating until it mixes each time properly.

- Combine flour, baking soda, salt and baking powder in a bowl before gently adding to the butter mixture.
- Once combined, fold into chocolate chips.
- Refrigerate for about 20 minutes if the dough is too soft before forming. Form into large discs (1/4 cup pasta each) and freeze or refrigerate until solid, at least 2 hours.
- Preheat oven to 350 degrees F.
- Bake the cookies for 11-12 minutes. DO NOT overcook. Cookies will appear in the oven. Let stand on the tray for at least 5 minutes to continue cooking and reaffirming. Enjoy!

Take your Notes Here and Create your Variant

PANERA BREAD COPYCAT CHICKEN NOODLE SOUP

Try this delicious recipe for chicken bread noodle soup. I think you will be amazed at how easy it is to prepare and how easy it is to prepare.

Total time: 25 minutes
Yield: 6 Servings

INGREDIENTS

- Chicken broth with 2 cans
- 2 boneless, skinless chicken breasts
- 2 cups chopped carrots
- 1 cup of egg pasta
- 2 cups of water
- 1/2 chopped onion
- 1 teaspoon thyme
- 1 teaspoon garlic salt (or use minced garlic)
- 2 cups diced celery
- 1 bay leaf
- Salt and pepper to taste

INSTRUCTIONS

- Cooking on the stove.
- Sprinkle a frying pan with olive oil.
- Start cooking carrots, onions, and celery for a few minutes.
- Chop the chicken and add it to the pan.
- Pour in the chicken stock and water.
- Add seasonings
- Bring to a boil and cook until chicken begins to crumble.
- Remove the chicken and the strips.

Back to the soup

- Add raw egg noodles and cook until cooked through.
- Serve with a loaf of good crusty bread.
- Kitchen crockpot:
- Put everything (except the noodles) in the clay pot.
- Simmer for 6-8 hours or 3-4 hours.
- Minutes before serving, remove chicken and shred.
- Back to the plate. Turn on the high pot and add the egg noodles.
- After about 30 minutes, the spaghetti will be cut and dinner will be served.

Take your Notes Here and Create your Variant

PANERA BREAD COPYCAT SPINACH AND CHEESE EGG SOUFFLE

Pillsbury Butter Flake's rising sandwiches are the foundation of these four cheese, bacon, spinach, and egg soufflés. The perfect recipe for breakfast or brunch!

Total time: 35 minutes.
Yield: 4 servings

INGREDIENTS

- 6 large eggs (hold one aside to brush the top of the crescent rolls)
- 1 roll 8-ounce Pillsbury butter flake tubes with butter
- 2 tablespoons of cream
- 2 tablespoons of milk
- 1/4 cup chopped Monterey Jack cheese
- 1/4 cup shredded cheddar cheese
- 3 tablespoons finely chopped fresh spinach
- 1/4 cup grated Asiago cheese
- 1 tablespoon of Parmesan
- 1/4 teaspoon of salt
- 4 slices of cooked and minced bacon

INSTRUCTIONS

- Preheat oven to 375 degrees.
- In a small microwave-safe bowl, combine 5 eggs, milk, cream, cheddar cheese, Monterey jack cheese, Parmesan, spinach, bacon, and salt. Mix well.
- Microwave this mixture for 30 seconds. Stir the mixture, then continue microwave cooking at 20-second intervals approximately 4-5 times. Your aim should be to get the egg mixture to thicken slightly. It will still be very fluid and raw, but the fact that it is only slightly thicker will help hold the growing mass when it folds.
- Unroll the growing dough and separate it into four rectangles. Press the perforated triangles together to create rectangles. Extend each rectangle until it is roughly a 6x6 square.
- Spray four copper or souffle pans (4-5 inches in diameter) with cooking spray. Arrange a crescent roll lying on each plate, with the edges hanging off the sides. Pour 1/3 cup of egg mixture over each growing mass.
- Sprinkle the Asiago cheese over the egg mixture, dividing the cheese between the 4 molds. Fold the growing dough over the egg mixture.
- Take the remaining egg and beat lightly on a small plate. Using a pastry brush, roll the egg over the dough on the crescent roll.
- Bake at 375 F for at least 20 minutes or until golden.

Take your Notes Here and Create your Variant

PANERA BREAD COPYCAT NAPA ALMOND CHICKEN SALAD

One of my favorites is the spicy and sweet Napa Chicken Salad with red grapes, almonds and crispy celery, all mixed with a creamy lemon dressing. It is a completely delicious and fresh tasting food that deserves to pass out.

Yield: 6 servings

INGREDIENTS

For the salad

- 1/2 cup of grapes, sliced
- 2 cups cooked chicken, chopped
- 1 stalk celery, chopped
- 2 green onions, sliced
- 1/2 teaspoon dried rosemary
- 2 tablespoons chopped fresh parsley
- 1/4 cup sliced almonds
- Salt and pepper to taste

For the dressing:

- 2 tablespoons sour cream

- 1/4 cup royal mayonnaise
- 1 teaspoon grated lemon zest
- 1 teaspoon of agave sweetener (or sweetener of your choice)
- 2 teaspoons of apple cider vinegar

INSTRUCTIONS

- In a large bowl, combine all the ingredients for the salad.
- In a small, separate plate, mix all ingredients together for flavor.
- Pour salad dressing and mix well. Refrigerate.
- Serve with a sandwich or as desired.

Take your Notes Here and Create your Variant

PANERA BREAD COPYCAT CRANBERRY ORANGE MUFFINS

Easy to Top Panera Muffin Recipe with fresh blueberries, orange zest and buttermilk.

Total time: 55 minutes
Yield: 6 cupcakes

INGREDIENTS

- 1 tablespoon of cornstarch
- 1 1/2 cups all-purpose flour
- 1/2 teaspoon of baking soda
- 1 1/2 teaspoons of baking powder
- 1/2 cup of vegetable oil
- 1/2 teaspoon salt
- 2 large eggs
- 2/3 cup granulated sugar
- 2 tablespoons of turbinado sugar
- 1/2 cup buttermilk
- 1 teaspoon of vanilla extract
- 1 1/2 cups fresh blueberries, divided
- 2 teaspoons of fresh orange peel

INSTRUCTIONS

- Preheat oven to about 375 degrees F. Line a muffin tin with 6 jumbo paper liners.

- In a medium bowl, mix dry ingredients such as flour, cornstarch, baking powder, baking soda, and salt until well combined.

- In a large bowl, mix the oil and sugar until well blended. Stir the eggs one at a time, then add the vanilla.

- Alternate by adding the flour and buttermilk mixture to the large mixing bowl to mix with the oil and sugar, stirring after each addition.

- Add the fresh orange zest and 1 cup blueberries. Pour the muffin dough into a prepared skillet.

- Press the remaining 1/2 cup of blueberries on top of each bun. Sprinkle the turbinado sugar over the muffins.

- Bake the muffins at 375 degrees F for about 25-30 minutes or until the golden brown edges appear and a toothpick inserted in the middle is clean.

- Cool slightly before removing the muffins from the pan and place them on the wire rack to finish cooling.

Take your Notes Here and Create your Variant

PANERA BREAD COPYCAT CHOPPED THAI GRILLED CHICKEN SALAD

This salad is a quick and easy recipe from Panera that has been lightened to eliminate some carbs and calories to make it keto-friendly and low carb. The salad is topped with homemade peanut dressing and made with juicy chicken thigh; you can use the chicken breast if you like.

Total time: 2 hours 35 minutes
Yield: 4 Servings

INGREDIENTS

Thai chicken marinade

- 1 teaspoon of ground or fresh ginger
- 1 pound boned butcher's chicken legs or chicken breast
- 1 teaspoon of sesame oil
- ½ tablespoon McCormick Grilled Chicken Dressing
- 1 tablespoon of soy sauce or liquid amino acids
- 1 teaspoon of rice wine vinegar
- 1 tablespoon Sriracha 1 tablespoon produces a delicate flavor, add more to suit your taste
- ½ tablespoon McCormick's Grill Mates barbecue seasoning
- Salt and pepper to taste

Salad

- 1/4 cup fresh green onions
- 1/4 cup fresh cilantro
- 2 tablespoons sliced peanuts or sunflower seeds
- 3 cups spinach or mixed vegetables
- 1 cup chopped cabbage
- Sesame seed topping

Thai peanut dressing

- 2 garlic cloves, minced
- 1/4 cup natural almond or peanut butter
- 2 tablespoons soy sauce or liquid amino acids
- 1 teaspoon of sesame oil
- 1 teaspoon of fish sauce
- 2 tablespoons brown sweetener
- 1 tablespoon of freshly squeezed lime juice
- 1/4 cup of water
- 1 tablespoon of apple cider vinegar

INSTRUCTIONS

For the Thai peanut dressing

- in a small bowl, add peanut butter. Sometimes natural peanut butter can be difficult to mix. If so, microwave it for 15-30 seconds to soften it.

- Add the other ingredients to the season in the bowl. Stir to combine until dressing becomes creamy.

Thai chicken salad

- Marinating chicken is recommended for optimal flavor and consistency. Add chicken in a sealable plastic bag with ginger, soy sauce, sesame oil, Sriracha, rice vinegar, barbecue seasoning, chicken seasoning, salt and pepper to taste.
- Shake the bag and make sure the chicken is completely covered. Store in the refrigerator for at least 2 hours overnight.
- Heat grill over medium-high heat (if you prefer to cook chicken, see cooking instructions below in Recipe Notes). Let the grill heat for 10 minutes.
- I like to spray my dishes with olive oil to avoid sticking.
- Add the chicken and cook for about 10-15 minutes until it reaches an internal temperature of 165 degrees, inverting it in half. Use a meat thermometer to test if you're ready.
- Remove the chicken from the grill. Let the chicken feet rest for 10 minutes before cutting them into strips.
- While the chicken rests, prepare the salad with spinach, cabbage, cilantro, green onion, and peanuts or sunflower seeds.
- Add the sliced chicken strips. Sprinkle on the Thai peanut sauce.

Take your Notes Here and Create your Variant

PANERA BREAD COPYCAT APPLE RAISIN COBBLESTONE MUFFINS

Panera's apple raisin cobblestone muffins are absolutely wonderful. You can make this from your home kitchen.

Total time: 1 hour
Yield: 12 Servings

INGREDIENTS

For Dough:

- 1 cup granulated sugar
- 4 eggs
- 2 cups skim milk, heated
- 2 packs (0.25 oz each) of fast yeast
- 1 teaspoon of kosher salt
- 7 cups flour, divided
- 4 ounces butter, melted

For the coating:

- 1 cup brown sugar
- 1 cup granulated sugar
- 3/4 cup butter, melted

- 1/4 cup cinnamon

For the filling:

- 1/2 cup golden raisins
- 1/2 cup raisins
- 2 apples, diced

For the icing:

- 2 tablespoons of milk
- 1 cup icing sugar

INSTRUCTIONS

- In a large bowl, mix the yeast with the hot milk. Add the eggs, sugar and salt. Continue mixing the melted butter and 3 cups of flour.
- Add remaining flour until it mixes properly, trying not to over-mix. Convert the pasta into a greased bowl, cover and let it grow to double its size.
- Line large muffin pans with linings or parchment paper. Put the melted butter in a bowl and combine the brown sugar, sugar and cinnamon in a separate bowl. Pinch 2 dumplings, 2 tablespoons in size, roll into a ball.
- Put the dough in melted butter, then in the mixture of sugar and cinnamon. Place at the bottom of the muffin cup. Repeat until you have 3 balls at the bottom of each cup.
- In a small bowl, mix the raisins with the apples. Put a tablespoon of filling on the dumplings. Repeat the

preparation of the dumplings adding 4 balls on top of each bun.

- Again, sprinkle with 1 tablespoon of apple filling/raisin. When all the muffins are ready, bake at 350 degrees for about 25 minutes.
- Remove and let cool. Mix together the icing sugar and milk in a small bowl. Sprinkle muffins and enjoy!

Take your Notes Here and Create your Variant

PANERA BREAD COPYCAT LEMON CHICKEN ORZO SOUP

This light and refreshing slow cooker recipe with lemon chicken and barley soup is an all year round delicacy and serves as a substitute for traditional chicken noodle soup!

Yield: 8 servings
Total time: 5 hours 45 minutes

INGREDIENTS

- 8 cups chicken broth
- 1 kg boneless, skinless chicken breast
- 3 carrots, chopped
- 1 small onion, chopped
- 1 bay leaf
- 2 tablespoons minced garlic
- 1/4 cup fresh parsley, chopped
- 1 teaspoon of black pepper
- 3/4 cup dried barley
- 2 lemons, zest and juice
- 2 tablespoons of dill
- 3 celery stalks, sliced

INSTRUCTIONS

- In a slow cooker, place the chicken breast, garlic, black pepper, parsley, dill, bay leaf, lemon zest, onion, carrots, and chicken stock. Cook 5 hours on top or 8 hours on the bottom
- Remove chicken and chop or cut. Put back into the slow cooker. Then add the barley paste, lemon juice, and celery. Cook for another 30 minutes.
- Try adjusting seasonings as needed and enjoy!

Take your Notes Here and Create your Variant

PANERA BREAD COPYCAT FUJI APPLE SALAD

A simple homemade version of Panera Bread Fuji Apple Salad with sliced chicken, fries, blue cheese, and more!

Total time: 15 minutes
Yield: 4 Servings

INGREDIENTS

- Panera Fuji Apple Vinaigrette dressing
- 3 cups thinly sliced cooked chicken breast
- 4 cups chopped washed and dried romaine lettuce
- 2-3 cups dried Seneca apples
- 2 cups of washed and dry rocket
- 1/2 red onion cut into thin slices
- 4 ripe tomatoes (on the smaller side), set aside and cut into 6 wedges
- 1/2 cup pecans (chopped if desired)
- 1/3 cup shredded Maytag or Gorgonzola blue cheese

INSTRUCTIONS

- Combine romaine lettuce, arugula, apple chips, sliced chicken breasts, tomato slices, sliced red onion, blue cheese

crumbs, and half walnuts in a large bowl.
- Drizzle with the desired amount of vinaigrette dressing and mix gently to combine. Serve and enjoy.

Take your Notes Here and Create your Variant

PANERA BREAD COPYCAT GREEN TEA

Get homemade green tea you love. Now you can make that Panera's green tea that you love at home with this simple recipe.

Total time: 11 minutes
Yield: 1 serving

INGREDIENTS

- Juice of one lemon
- 4 teaspoons of honey
- 6 green tea bags
- Fresh mint (optional)

INSTRUCTIONS

- Boil six cups of water.
- Add green tea bags.
- Remove from heat and let it cool down.
- Microwave the honey for at least 20 seconds and mix the honey in the green tea.
- Add the lemon juice.
- Garnish with fresh mint.

TAKE YOUR NOTES HERE AND CREATE YOUR VARIANT

PANERA BREAD COPYCAT HUMMUS BOWL

Hummus Bowl is a high-fiber, low-calorie, healthy salad for every meal. You can make it at home with this recipe.

Total time: 25 minutes
Yield: 4 servings

INGREDIENTS

- 2 teaspoons of olive oil
- ½ teaspoon of paprika
- 2 large chicken breasts
- ½ teaspoon poultry dressing (a combination of dried basil, marjoram, rosemary, sage, oregano, and thyme)
- 12 ounces baby spinach leaves
- ½ English cucumber, thinly sliced
- 2 Roma tomatoes, diced
- ⅓ cup chopped cilantro to season
- 2 lemons, cut in half
- 1 small red onion, thinly sliced
- Salt and pepper

For the cilantro-jalapeño hummus

- 2 garlic cloves, minced
- 1 can of rinsed and drained, skinned low-sodium chickpeas
- 3 tablespoons of fresh lime juice
- 2 tablespoons of tahini
- ½ cup canned cilantro leaves, chopped
- ¼ teaspoon of cumin
- 4 tablespoons of water
- ½ teaspoon of salt
- 2 tablespoons of olive oil
- ½ chopped fresh jalapeño

INSTRUCTIONS

For the hummus

- Combine all of the ingredients in a food processor and smoothies until smooth.
- Transfer the mixture to a container and refrigerate until necessary.
- Combine the paprika and chicken dressing and reserve. To make chicken, pound the chicken breasts with an even thickness. Season both sides with pepper, paprika, salt and poultry dressing
- Heat the oil over medium heat. Add chicken breasts and cook at least 10 minutes or until cooked through. Remove on a plate to cool. Then cut into thin slices.
- Put 2 or 3 cups of spinach in a large salad bowl. Garnish with tomatoes, cucumbers, red onions, grilled chicken slices (1/2 large chicken breast for salad), half a lemon and a ball

of cilantro and jalapeño hummus, and a generous pinch of chopped cilantro. Enjoy!

Take your Notes Here and Create your Variant

PANERA BREAD COPYCAT HONEY WALNUT PANERA CREAM CHEESE

Prepare your favorite cream cheese at home to spread on your favorite baked goods.

Yield: 4-6 Servings

INGREDIENTS

- 1/2 teaspoon of vanilla extract
- 4 ounces cream cheese
- 3 tablespoons of finely chopped walnuts
- 2 tablespoons of honey
- 1/2 teaspoon of cinnamon

INSTRUCTIONS

- Combine all the ingredients except walnuts in a bowl.
- Beat with a medium speed manual electric mixer until everything is incorporated and the cream cheese becomes "soft."
- Mix the nuts with a spatula or spoon. Enjoy!

Take your Notes Here and Create your Variant

PANERA BREAD COPYCAT ASIAGO CHEESE BREAD

A crispy crust, smooth inside with a fantastic taste of Asiago cheese. So good with soup, salad or in a sandwich.

Total time 1 hour and 20 minutes.
Yield: 20 Servings

INGREDIENTS

- 1 packet of Superior Platinum Red Star baking powder (2 1/4 teaspoons)
- 3 1/4 cups all-purpose flour
- 1 teaspoon of granulated sugar
- 1 1/2 teaspoons of salt
- 1 1/4 cups milk
- 1/4 teaspoon black pepper
- 1 1/2 cups grated Asiago cheese (broken)
- 2 butter spoons

For brushing on top:

- 1 large egg, beaten

INSTRUCTIONS

- In a food processor bowl, combine 1 1/2 cups of flour, yeast, sugar, salt, and pepper. Put the milk in a microwave-safe container.

- Add the butter. Heat the milk to about 120 degrees so that the butter begins to melt. Make sure the temperature is right, so it is hot enough to activate the yeast, but don't kill it.

- Combine the flour mixture and milk mixture and mix on low speed using the spoon attachment until smooth. Add 1 1/4 cups of grated cheese and stir just until combined.

- Gradually add 1 1/4 cups of flour to make a smooth dough. Knead in the food processor with the dough hook for 5 minutes.

- Spray a bowl with cooking spray. Add the dough to the bowl, then flip the dough upside down, so the cooking spray covers both sides of the dough.

- Cover the bowl and let the dough rise in a warm place until it doubles (anywhere between 1-2 hours).

- After folding the dough, tap it and make two loaves. Place the loaves on a sprayed baking sheet.

- Cover the loaves and let them rise until they double, which will take 30 to 45 minutes.

- Preheat oven to 375 degrees.

- Make 3-4 cuts on top of the loaves with a serrated knife. Brush the top of the loaves with the beaten egg, then sprinkle with the remaining cheese. Cook for 30-35 minutes until lightly browned.

Take your Notes Here and Create your Variant

PANERA BREAD COPYCAT SOBA NOODLE BROTH BOWL WITH CHICKEN

I really like these broth bowls that I had to immediately recreate it at home.

Total time: 1 hour and 15 minutes.
Yield: 4 servings

INGREDIENTS

- ⅓ cup of herb marinade and lemon pepper (link below)
- 2 boneless, skinless chicken breasts
- ½ a small yellow onion
- 2 teaspoons sesame oil
- 2 tablespoons soy sauce
- ½ cup shitake sliced mushrooms or cremini work well
- 2 teaspoons of Sriracha and more to taste
- 1 teaspoon of brown sugar
- 4 cups chicken broth
- 1 medium peeled carrot and julienne
- ½ cup yellow miso
- 2 cups of water
- ¼ cup red cabbage, thinly sliced
- 8 ounces of soba paste

- 1 cup freshly packed fresh spinach
- ½ cup chopped Napa cabbage
- 1 teaspoon of chopped cilantro to decorate
- ½ teaspoon sesame seeds

INSTRUCTIONS

- In a sealable container, add chicken and marinade and mix to coat. Set aside to marinate for about 30 minutes (or overnight).
- Place the chicken on a preheated grill or fry and cook, basting with the remaining marinade for 8-10 minutes aside. Once cooked through the chicken, they will be firm, opaque, and if you hit them with a fork, the juices will flow clear.
- Remove from the heat and reserve before cutting. Meanwhile, heat oil over medium heat and brown onions and mushrooms until they begin to brown and caramelize, about 6 minutes.
- Add soy sauce, brown sugar, and Sriracha until well blended.
- Add carrots and cook for another minute before mixing broth, water and miso. Cook, stirring gently until the miso is completely melted.
- Add cabbage and soba noodles and cook until noodles are tender for about 5 minutes.
- Mix spinach and ladle in individual bowls.
- Slice the chicken and top it garnished with sesame and cilantro seeds to serve.

TAKE YOUR NOTES HERE AND CREATE YOUR VARIANT

PANERA BREAD COPYCAT CHICKEN CAESAR SANDWICH

Prepare your favorite Panera chicken Caesar sandwich at home to spread the love with your family.

Total time: 40 minutes
Yield: 4 servings

INGREDIENTS

- 1 loaf Panera sourdough bread
- 2 half boneless skinless chicken breast
- 2-4 peeled garlic cloves
- 2 spoons of olive oil
- 1 small head romaine lettuce, cut into 1-inch slices
- 8 slices of sourdough bread
- 1/4 cup grated parmesan
- 1/3 Caesar salad dressing prepared in the cup
- 1 tomato, cut into wedges (optional)
- Red onion, cut in half
- Freshly ground pepper

INSTRUCTIONS

- Chop 2 or 4 cloves of garlic (4 is great if you love garlic) and set them aside. Cut the chicken into 1/4 inch slices. Heat the olive oil in a pan and fry the garlic for 30 seconds or until the aroma is released. Add chicken and brown until cooked through, 3 to 5 minutes. Season to taste with pepper. Turn off the heat and set it aside.

- Grill or broil bread until lightly toasted, about 1 minute per side.
- In a bowl, combine the romaine lettuce, salad dressing, Parmesan, red onion, and chicken. Season to taste with pepper. Place 4 slices of toast, add remaining toast and serve with tomatoes on the side if desired. Makes four servings.
- Picnic packing instructions: sauté the chicken with garlic and cool slightly. Pack in a plastic container and refrigerate.
- Put the toast in a plastic bag and pack it. (Do not seal the bag or the toast will be soaked.)
- Put the lettuce in a large, closed bowl. Pour the salad dressing into a plastic container. Pour the cheese into a plastic container. Pack the red onion and tomatoes, if used, in a plastic bag.
- Refrigerate everything except toast until transport to the picnic. Pack everything except toast in the refrigerator with ice or cold packs. (Package of toasts at room temperature).

Take your Notes Here and Create your Variant

PANERA BREAD COPYCAT SPINACH AND ARTICHOKE SOUFFLE

Prepare your favorite spinach and artichoke souffle at home. It easy and delicious!

Total time: 50 minutes
Yield: 4 servings

INGREDIENTS

- 2 tablespoons unsalted butter
- 1 cup of whole milk
- 2 spoons of all-purpose flour
- 1/4 teaspoon black pepper
- 1/2 teaspoon of salt
- 3 big eggs
- 1/2 cup spinach with artichoke sauce
- 1/4 cup grated Roman cheese
- 1/2 grated bowl of Monterey jack cheese
- 1/4 teaspoon minced chili flakes
- 1/2 teaspoon granulated garlic
- 1 frozen puff pastry, thawed
- 2. 3 chop hot sauce

INSTRUCTIONS

- Preheat the oven to about 425 degrees F. Grease 4 round pans with cooking spray and place on a baking sheet, set aside.
- Put a saucepan over medium heat with the butter. Once melted, beat the flour and cook for about 30 seconds. Add milk and cook, frequently stirring, until sauce thickens. Season with a pinch of pepper and salt. Remove from heat and let cool slightly.
- In a large bowl, mix the spinach and artichoke sauce, eggs, cold milk sauce, Monterey Jack cheese, Roman cheese, garlic, pepper flakes, and hot sauce until well combined.
- Discard the puff pastry and cut the sheet into four squares. Place a square on each mold, pressing down and up on the sides of each mold. Divide the souffle mixture between the molds.
- Cook until puffed up and turns deep golden brown, about 25-30 minutes. Remove from the oven and let cool slightly before serving.

Take your Notes Here and Create your Variant

PANERA BREAD COPYCAT BACON TURKEY BRAVO SANDWICH

Prepare your favorite bacon turkey bravo sandwich at home.

Total time: 10 minutes
Yield: 1 serving

INGREDIENTS

- 1/2 cup of tomato sauce
- 1 mayonnaise cup
- 1/2 teaspoon dried mustard
- 2 tablespoons lemon juice, freshly squeezed
- 1 sprinkle with Tabasco sauce
- 1 teaspoon Worcestershire sauce

Sandwich

- 1 Romaine lettuce leaf
- 2 slices of bread with tomato and basil (or another hearty favorite)
- 4 ounces thinly sliced smoked turkey breast
- 3 tomato slices (1/4 inch thick)
- 2 slices of bacon, crispy cooked
- 1 slice of smoked gouda cheese

INSTRUCTIONS

Dressing:

- Combine all ingredients in a small bowl and mix well.
- Refrigerate.
- This makes 1 3/4 cups and will stay in the refrigerator for a long time.

Sandwich:

- Spread 2 tablespoons of seasoning on one of the bread slices (we put it on both sides).
- On a slice of bread, a layer of lettuce, tomato, turkey, gouda and bacon.
- Top with the second slice of bread and serve.

Take your Notes Here and Create your Variant

PANERA BREAD COPYCAT CREAM CHEESE POTATO SOUP

Prepare your favorite cream cheese potato soup at home.

Total time: 1 hour
Yield: 4-6 servings

INGREDIENTS

- 4 cups peeled and diced potatoes
- 4 cups chicken broth
- 1/4 teaspoon white pepper
- 1/2 teaspoon salt seasoning
- 1 (8 ounces) package cream cheese, cut into pieces
- 1/4 teaspoon ground red pepper

INSTRUCTIONS

- Combine broth, potatoes and spices.
- Boil over medium heat until the potatoes are tender.
- Break some potatoes to release the starch to thicken.
- Reduce heat to low.
- Add the cream cheese.
- Heat, frequently stirring, until cheese is melted.

Take your Notes Here and Create your Variant

PANERA BREAD COPYCAT FRONTEGA CHICKEN PANINI

Panera's Frontega chicken panini is just another of my favorite Panera menu items.

Yield: 4 servings

INGREDIENTS

- 1 hot pepper in marinade sauce + 1 or 2 teaspoons of sauce
- 1/4 cup mayonnaise
- 2 chicken breasts (12-14 ounces total), cooked and minced
- 4 focaccia (or 1 focaccia bread, quartered)
- Extra virgin olive oil or non-stick spray
- 1 tomato, sliced
- 8 ounces mozzarella ball, sliced
- 10-12 fresh chopped basil leaves
- 1/2 small red onion, sliced

INSTRUCTIONS

- Add mayonnaise, chili pepper, and marinade sauce to a bowl for a mini food processor, then continue until smooth. Alternatively, finely chop the pepper, then mix with the mayonnaise sauce.

- Spread chipotle mayonnaise on top and bottom of sandwiches, then spread over shredded chicken, tomato, red onion, mozzarella, and fresh basil.
- Press the sandwiches press over medium-high heat until the cheese melts and the bread is crisp. Serve immediately

Take your Notes Here and Create your Variant

PANERA BREAD COPYCAT ORANGE SCONES

Prepare your favorite orange scones at home to spread on your favorite Panera menu item.

Total time: 35 minutes
Yield: 12 serving (12 large buns)

INGREDIENTS

For the scones:

- 1/2 cup granulated sugar
- 1 1/2 cup all-purpose flour
- 2 teaspoons of baking powder
- 1/4 cup plain Greek yogurt
- 1/4 teaspoon kosher salt
- 1 large egg
- 6 tablespoons unsalted butter, diced, softened
- 1/4 cup orange juice
- 1 teaspoon grated orange zest
- 1/2 teaspoonful of orange extract

For the icing:

- 1 teaspoon grated orange zest
- 2 tablespoons of orange juice
- 1 cup icing sugar

INSTRUCTIONS

- For the muffins, combine the flour, sugar, salt, and yeast in a large bowl. Add the butter. Stir using the mixer blade of an electric mixer until it looks like thick crumbs.
- Add egg, yogurt, orange juice, orange extract, and orange zest. Fully combine
- On a large baking sheet with parchment paper, form the dough into a large rectangle (about 9 inches x 7 inches by 1/2 inch thick). Use your hands to rub the dough; it will be sticky. Sprinkle with flour to make it viable.
- Using a large knife or pizza cutter, cut the dough in half and then cut it into thirds, creating six rectangles.
- Cut each rectangle in half to create 2 triangles. You will have a total of 12 triangles. Do not separate them on the baking sheet yet!
- Bake at 350 degrees for 25 minutes. Remove from the oven and carefully cut the triangles. Separate and return to the oven for another 10-15 minutes. Remove and cool completely before frosting.
- For the icing, mix the icing sugar, orange zest, and orange juice. Put ice on each chilled bun, let stand, about 15 minutes. Store in an airtight container for up to 4 days. Enjoy!

TAKE YOUR NOTES HERE AND CREATE YOUR VARIANT

PANERA BREAD COPYCAT ASIAN SESAME CHICKEN SALAD

Asian Sesame Chicken Salad are good for dinner. You can make this at home and enjoy it with the rest of your family.

Total time: 30 minutes
Yield: 1 serving

INGREDIENTS

Salad

- Canola oil, for frying
- 2 wonton wrappers
- 1 tablespoon of sesame seeds
- 4 cups small pieces romaine lettuce, packaged
- 2 tablespoons sliced almonds
- 3 ounces boneless, skinless, grilled and thinly sliced chicken breast in an injury
- 1 tablespoon chopped fresh cilantro

Asian sesame dressing

- 1/8 cup toasted sesame oil
- 1/8 cup rice wine vinegar

- 1/2 teaspoon toasted sesame seeds
- 1 tablespoon soy sauce
- 1/3 cup rapeseed or vegetable oil
- 1/2 teaspoon minced red pepper flakes

INSTRUCTIONS

- Preheat, oven to 350 degrees F.
- To prepare the Wonton strips, cut the Wonton strips into 1/4 inch strips. In a deep skillet, pour canola oil to a depth of 2-3 inches. Heat oil to 365 degrees F.
- Carefully place wonton slices in hot oil and fry for about 30 seconds, or until crisp and golden. Remove with a perforated spoon and drain on a paper towel.
- Arrange the almonds in a single layer on a baking sheet. Toast in the oven for 5 minutes, mix the nuts, then toast for another 5 minutes or until golden brown. Remove from the pan to cool.
- To make Asian sesame dressing, combine all ingredients except canola oil in a medium bowl with wire whisk.
- Once the ingredients combine, slowly pour in the oil while whisking to form an emulsion.
- To make the salad, mix the lettuce, cilantro, wonton strips, chicken, and seasonings (amount to taste) in large bowl until combined.
- Put the mixture on a serving plate. Sprinkle with sesame and almond seeds and serve.

Take your Notes Here and Create your Variant

PANERA BREAD COPYCAT BROWN BETTY

Prepare your favorite Panera brown betty at home and enjoy it with your family.

Total time: 60 minutes
Yield: 8 servings

INGREDIENTS

- 8 tablespoons of butter
- 1 cup breadcrumbs
- 1/2 teaspoon of cinnamon
- 1 cup of white sugar
- 1 teaspoon of vanilla extract
- 6 apples or pears or peaches, peeled, carrots, and chopped
- 1/2 teaspoon of nutmeg
- 2 beaten eggs
- 1/2 cup brown sugar

INSTRUCTIONS

- Generously baking butter. Mix the spices with fruit and brown sugar. Put in the pan.
- In a small bowl, beat the eggs with the vanilla. In a separate

bowl, with a fork, mix the breadcrumbs with the white sugar.
- Cover the fruit with the breadcrumb mixture and pour the melted butter over the breadcrumbs, carefully covering. Bake at 350 ° F for 30 to 40 minutes.

Take your Notes Here and Create your Variant

HARVEST TURKEY SALAD WITH CHERRY VINAIGRETTE

Prepare your favorite Harvest turkey salad with vinaigrette at home.

Total time: 40 minutes
Yield: 8 servings

INGREDIENTS

Harvest turkey salad

- 1/2 bag of romaine lettuce cut into small pieces
- 1 large spring/field mix
- 1 cup walnuts or roasted walnuts
- 8 ounces of feta cheese we prefer gorgonzola feta cheese
- 2 large unpeeled pears
- 1 cup dried cherries
- 1-2 cups grilled chicken or sliced turkey breast
- Lemon juice (optional)

Cherry vinaigrette

- 1 tablespoon. sugar
- 1/4 cup balsamic vinegar

- 1/4 cup cherry jam Smucker
- 1 clove garlic, minced
- 1/4 cup olive oil
- 1/4 cup red wine vinegar
- Freshly ground black pepper to taste
- Salt to taste

INSTRUCTIONS

Harvest turkey salad

- Place the lettuces in a wide salad bowl.
- Add the dried cherries.
- Peel and cut pears and shellfish in a small bowl of lemon juice to prevent discoloration.
- Add other salad ingredients.
- Toast walnuts or walnuts in the oven or toaster at 350 for about 5-10 minutes.
- Add roasted walnuts on top.
- Sprinkle with feta or gorgonzola.
- Add the chicken or turkey breast to the grill, sliced, or diced.
- Keep in the refrigerator until ready to serve.
- Serve with cherry vinaigrette.

Vinaigrette cherry

- In a small saucepan over medium heat, combine the balsamic vinegar, sugar, and garlic and simmer, frequently stirring to

dissolve the sugar.
- Simmer the mixture, uncovered, until it is halved, about 10 minutes.
- Add cherry preserves and cook 1 minute more.
- Remove from heat and allow to cool to room temperature.
- Whisk in red wine vinegar followed by canola oil.
- Spice with salt and pepper.
- Set aside. Serve over the turkey salad collection.

Take your Notes Here and Create your Variant

PANERA BREAD COPYCAT CHIPOTLE CHICKEN AVOCADO MELT

This chipotle chicken and avocado melt is a dash of the Panera bread sandwich, complete with focaccia, smoked gouda, and roasted red peppers!

Total Time: 30 minutes
Yield: 4 servings

INGREDIENTS

- 1 chicken breast
- 1 loaf of bread
- 4 slices of smoked gouda
- 1 avocado, sliced
- 1/4 cup roasted red bell peppers, sliced

Chipotle mayo

- 1/2 chopped chili
- 1 tablespoon adobo sauce (from a can of chipotles)
- 1/3 cup light mayonnaise

INSTRUCTIONS

- Add chicken breast in a large saucepan with boiling water and cook for 15-20 minutes or until the internal temperature of chicken reaches 165 F.
- Remove from water, then destroy chicken and season with salt and pepper.
- Cut the focaccia in half lengthwise if necessary. Mix the ingredients for the chipotle mayonnaise, then spread a little over a spoon over half the focaccia.
- Top with 1/4 chicken, about 1 tablespoon roasted red pepper, 1/4 avocado, and a slice of cheese.
- Top with remaining slice of focaccia, then add to a skillet over medium heat. Put the lid on and cook for 3-4 minutes until the cheese has melted. Serve and enjoy!

Take your Notes Here and Create your Variant

PANERA BREAD COPYCAT MODERN GREEK SALAD

This modern Greek salad is one of my favorite Panera bread salad! It's easy to make at home and great for a healthy lunch!

Total time: 10 minutes
Yield: 2 servings

INGREDIENTS

- 1 tablespoon of red wine vinegar
- 2 tablespoons of olive oil
- ¼ teaspoon garlic powder
- ¼ teaspoon dried oregano
- ¼ teaspoon onion powder
- 2 cups of cabbage, destemmed and massaged (see note)
- 2 cups chopped romaine lettuce
- ¼ cup cooked quinoa
- ¼ cup crumbled feta cheese
- 2 tablespoons minced cucumber
- ¼ cup sliced almonds
- Pinch of salt

INSTRUCTIONS

- Whisk with olive oil, red wine vinegar, oregano, garlic powder, onion powder and salt. Set aside.
- In a large bowl, combine the romaine lettuce and black cabbage.
- Top with feta cheese, quinoa, sliced almonds, and cucumber.
- Sprinkle with seasoning and divide evenly into two bowls.

Take your Notes Here and Create your Variant

PANERA BREAD MENU

BAKED EGG SOUFFLES

Spinach & Bacon Souffle

Ham & Swiss Baked Egg Souffle

Four Cheese Souffle

Spinach & Artichoke Souffle

SANDWICHES

Avocado, Egg White & Spinach Breakfast Power Sandwich

Sausage, Egg & Cheese On Ciabatta

Turkey Sausage, Egg White & Spinach Breakfast Power Sandwich

Mediterranean Egg White Sandwich

Steak & Egg On Everything Bagel

Asiago Cheese Bagel with Bacon, Egg & Cheese

Ham, Egg & Cheese Breakfast Power Sandwich

Parfaits, Fruit Cups and Oatmeal

Steel Cut Oatmeal with Apple Chips & Pecans

Power Almond Quinoa Oatmeal

Fresh Fruit Cup

Bacon, Egg & Cheese On Ciabatta

Steel Cut Oatmeal with Strawberries & Pecans

Egg & Cheese On Grilled Ciabatta

Strawberry Parfait

SOUPS AND MAC & CHEESE

Mac & Cheese

Bistro French Onion Soup

Low-Fat Garden Vegetable Soup with Pesto

Baked Potato Soup

Low-Fat Chicken Noodle Soup

Turkey Chili

Broccoli Cheddar Soup

Vegetarian Creamy Tomato Soup

Bistro French Onion Soup

Baked Potato Soup

SALADS

Green Goddess Cobb Salad with Chicken

Fuji Apple Salad with Chicken

Whole Beet & Citrus Salad

Half Beet & Citrus Salad

Romaine & Kale Caesar Salad with Chicken

Spicy Thai Salad with Chicken

Chinese Citrus Cashew Salad with Chicken

Modern Greek Salad with Quinoa

Caesar Salad with Chicken

BBQ Salad with Chicken

Seasonal Greens Salad

Caesar Salad

Fresh Fruit Cup

Greek Salad

PANINI & SANDWICHES

Chipotle Chicken Avocado Melt

Roasted Turkey & Caramelized Kale Panini

Roasted Turkey, Apple & Cheddar Sandwich

Roasted Turkey & Avocado BLT

Steak & White Cheddar Panini

Frontega Chicken Panini

The Italian Sandwich

Bacon Turkey Bravo Sandwich

Steak & Arugula Sandwich

Ham & Swiss Sandwich

Napa Almond Chicken Salad Sandwich

Mediterranean Veggie Sandwich

Classic Grilled Cheese

Tuna Salad Sandwich

Turkey Sandwich

ONE FLATBREAD

Tomato Mozzarella Flatbread

BBQ Chicken Flatbread

TWO FLATBREADS

BBQ Chicken Flatbread

Tomato Mozzarella Flatbread

PASTA

Tortellini Alfredo Pasta

Chicken Tortellini Alfredo

PASTA MEAL

Chicken Tortellini Alfredo with Salad

Tortellini Alfredo Pasta with Salad

Tortellini Alfredo Pasta with Soup

Chicken Tortellini Alfredo with Flatbread

Tortellini Alfredo Pasta with Panini & Sandwich

Chicken Tortellini Alfredo with Soup

Tortellini Alfredo Pasta with Flatbread

Chicken Tortellini Alfredo with Panini & Sandwich

BAKERY

Bagels
Asiago Bagel

Cinnamon Crunch Bagel

Blueberry Bagel

Plain Bagel

Cinnamon Swirl Bagel

Everything Bagel

Sprouted Grain Bagel Flat

Chocolate Chip Bagel

Sesame Bagel

Whole Grain Bagel

French Toast Bagel

SPREADS

Honey Walnut Cream Cheese

Plain Cream Cheese

Reduced Fat Cream Cheese

Hazelnut Cream Cheese

Wild Blueberry Cream Cheese

Reduced-Fat Roasted Veg

Preserves

Chive and Onion Cream Cheese

Plain Cream Cheese Tub

Peanut Butter

Hazelnut Cream Cheese Tub

Honey Walnut Cream Cheese Tub

Reduced-Fat Roasted Veg Tub

Reduced Fat Cream Cheese Tub

Chive and Onion Cream Cheese Tub

Wild Blueberry Cream Cheese Tub

PASTRIES & SWEETS

Bear Claw

Cinnamon Roll

Chocolate Pastry

Pecan Braid

Cherry Pastry

Cheese Pastry

Butter Croissant

Cinnamon Crumb Coffee Cake Slice

Pecan Roll

Cobblestone

COOKIES & BROWNIES

Chocolate Chip Cookie

Tulip Cookie

Oatmeal Raisin with Berries Cookie

Raspberry Almond Thumbprint Cookie

Candy Cookie

Petite Cookies

Coconut Macaroon

Kitchen Sink Cookie

Chocolate Brownie

Shortbread Cookie

Gluten Conscious Triple Chocolate Cookie with Walnuts

MUFFINS & MUFFIES

Pumpkin Muffin

Blueberry Muffin with Fresh Blueberries

Apple Crunch Muffin

Cranberry Orange Muffin

Pumpkin Muffie

Chocolate Chip Muffie

SCONES

Cinnamon Crunch Scone

Mini Scones Variety Pack

Orange Scone

Caramel Apple Thumbprint Scone

Wild Blueberry Scone

BREAD

Cinnamon Raisin Swirl Loaf

French Baguette

Sourdough Bread

Asiago Cheese

Tomato Basil Loaf

Whole Grain Pan Loaf

Honey Wheat Loaf

Ciabatta Loaf

Rye Pan Loaf

Classic White Bread

Country

Sea Salt Focaccia Loaf

Asiago Cheese Focaccia

Hoagie Roll

Sesame Semolina Bread

Sprouted Whole Grain Roll

Soft Dinner Roll

SIDES AND SPREADS - SIDES

Chips

French Baguette

Soft Dinner Roll

Apple

Strawberry Squeezable Yogurt

Sprouted Whole Grain Roll

Fresh Fruit Cup

Blueberry Squeezable Yogurt

Strawberry Parfait

Banana

PANERA KID'S BEVERAGES

Horizon Reduced Fat Organic Chocolate Milk

Horizon Reduced Fat Organic White Milk

Coffee, Hot Tea and Hot Chocolate

Organic Apple Juice

Hot Tea

Hot Coffee

Hot Chocolate with Chocolate Chip

Iced Coffee

ESPRESSO BAR

Caffe Latte

Caramel Latte

Caffe Mocha

Chai Tea Latte

Iced Caramel Latte

Espresso

Cappuccino

Iced Chai Tea Latte

Iced Caffe Mocha

Iced Caffe Latte

ICED TEAS & LEMONADE

Lemonade

Iced Tea

Iced Green Tea

FROZEN DRINKS AND SMOOTHIES

Low Fat Mango Smoothie

Green Passion Power Smoothie

Carrot Pineapple Power Smoothie

Low-Fat Strawberry Banana Smoothie

Fat-Free Superfruit Power Smoothie

Strawberry Smoothie

Frozen Caramel

Frozen Mocha

MILK & JUICE

Organic Apple Juice

Orange Juice

Horizon Reduced Fat Organic Chocolate Milk

Horizon Reduced Fat Organic White Milk

SOFT & BOTTLED DRINKS

Bottled Water

Soda

San Pellegrino Orange

San Pellegrino Sparkling Water

Bottled Passion Fruit Papaya Green Tea

Joia Grapefruit Soda

Spindrift Raspberry Lime Seltzer

Spindrift Lemon Seltzer

Purity Organic Strawberry Paradise Juice

Panera Bottled Lemonade

SOUPS

Turkey Chili

Ten Vegetable Soup

Baked Potato Soup

New England Clam Chowder

Low-Fat Chicken Noodle Soup

Vegetarian Creamy Tomato Soup

Broccoli Cheddar Soup

Bistro French Onion Soup

Cream of Chicken & Wild Rice Soup

CONCLUSION

Panera Bread is one of my favorite restaurants when I want something light and fresh. They offer sandwiches, soups and other really delicious treats that would make you swear they were homemade. Panera Copycat bread recipes are the perfect way to get those comforting meals right at home.

This Panera bread copycat recipes bring our home to life. From now on, you can make your favorite Panera's delicacies at home. From the creamy broccoli cheddar soup to the incredibly delicious Black Bean Soup. Enjoy the best that Panera Bread has to offer by recreating them yourself with the help of these rich Panera Bread Copycat Recipes!

Patty Stewart

APPRECIATION

We sincerely appreciate your purchase of our book that reveals useful information on 40 different Panera Bread recipes that you can try at home. We hope you love them!

Made in the USA
Coppell, TX
22 November 2021

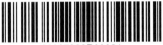